A Guide to Alternative Chiropractic Technique:
How to Keep Your Healing Practice From Hurting You

Written by Danielle Trego Finden, D.C.
Photography by Stephanie Hynes
Pagination & Graphic Design by Mary Trego and Michelle Sallee
Copyright 2014 by Danielle Trego Finden, D.C.
ISBN: 978-0-9904239-3-5

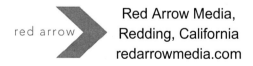

Red Arrow Media,
Redding, California
redarrowmedia.com

All rights reserved

No part of this manuscript may be used or reproduced in any matter whatsoever without written permission from the publisher, except in the case of brief quotations embodied in critical articles and reviews. For more information, please contact customercare@redarrowmedia.com

FIRST EDITION

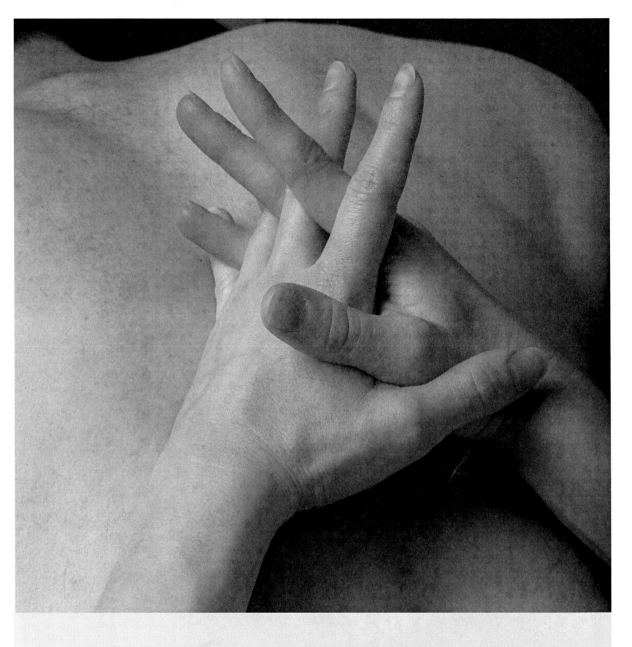

A Guide to Alternative Chiropractic Technique:
How to Keep Your Healing Practice from Hurting You

Danielle Trego Finden, D.C.

TABLE OF CONTENTS

Endorsements i
Acknowledgements ii
Preface iii

Chapter 1 Cervical and Cervicothoracic Junction 1
    Ah, Flex It - Now Push It Real Good 2
    Take a Seat 4
    Double Fist Pump.................................... 8
    Iron Cross... 10

Chapter 2 Thoracic 12
    Everyone Needs a Hug 13
    Tuck & Tumble 18
    Knife Thrower....................................... 20
    Don't Pop The Collar 22

Chapter 3 Thoracolumbar Junction...................... 24
    Shoot for the Moon................................ 26
    Ring 'em Out 28

Chapter 4 Lumbar and Pelvis.............................. 32
    The Lumbar Lambada 34
    The Elvis 38

Chapter 5 Extraspinal 41
    Hitchhiking Together.............................. 42
    Thumb Wrestling 44
    Bunny Hop 46
    Mini Hop.. 48

Chapter 6 Adjusting The Overweight Patient, The Very Tall Patient, & The Very Muscular Patient........ 50
    Fire Hydrant 54
    Wrestling Match 58
    No-Neck Nunchucks 62

Appendix 65
References 67

ENDORSEMENTS

"As a smaller chiropractor, I am delighted to see a book that provides optional adjustment approaches by a seasoned DC. During my 22 years in practice, I have also had to modify several adjustments after finding it painful to use the techniques I learned in school. I have also had to help students of varied sizes, strengths, and abilities learn to competently adjust. Dr. Finden's presentation of optional techniques is fun, clear, and profound in their simplicity. The images are high quality and make it easy to understand the technique that she is describing. This is a book that I will recommend to all chiropractors regardless of body type. Thank you!"

Anne Spicer, D.C., DACCP
Associate Professor Bloomington Natural Care Center
Northwestern Health Sciences University

"I had the great privilege of being mentored by Dr. Finden as an intern at her clinic while she was creating this book. Each technique is uniquely created, carefully articulated, and successful when applied to the patient. I am still reveling in all of the practical wisdom and knowledge I received from her and this book. I am currently in a post-doctoral residency at the VA Medical Center and daily utilizing these adjustment modifications in order to provide the necessary care to patients. I find myself teaching other interns many 'nuggets of gold' I received from Dr. Finden. She is remarkable, and this book is just the beginning! I highly recommend it to all new practitioners specializing in manual manipulative care."

Kate Craig, D.C.
Post-doctoral resident VA Medical Center St. Louis, MO

"Dr. Finden has given us such a gift! Her descriptions and the amazing photography enlighten and put into words the finesse and adaptations many of us learn when having to create a style that works for our body size. She opens the door for the smaller-framed chiropractor to become empowered in their art! I wish this book was available while I was in school! Thank you Dr. Finden!"

Lona Cook, D.C.
Author of Just Tell me Where to Start

"Dr. Finden's manual helps protect your most important asset: your ability to work. As a female chiropractor who works with elite athletes, I will definitely be including some of these tips in my practice to help me stay injury free. I highly recommend Dr. Finden's manual to any practitioner—from the novice to the experienced chiropractor—looking to protect his or her body from injuries in their wellness practice."

Nicole Hamel, D.C.
Team Chiropractor for the Minnesota TwinStars

ACKNOWLEDGEMENTS

Kate Craig, [intern extraordinaire] for helping me identify and articulate the techniques that I use in practice every day, which I often overlook as unique. And for sharing in my passion of all things pumpkin flavored.

My supportive [handsome] husband. I obviously could not have written this book without you washing all the dishes and folding endless amounts of laundry.

Molly Meri Robinson Nicol, for being a pioneer for the chiropractic profession and representing all of us worldwide with grace and the highest level of professionalism. And for participating in extreme sports to entertain my husband while I attend continuing education conferences!

My patients, for enabling me to develop these techniques in clinical practice with confidence and for giving me awesome nicknames like "chiro-ninja."

My publisher, for their patience and enthusiasm through the process and for making it as easy as possible for me to share my passion and experience in chiropractic practice.

Stephanie Hynes, for the beautiful images and amazing anatomy synonyms that keep me laughing.

Dan Galvin, Megan Eiselt, Jason Welke, and Joe Richter for graciously modeling and allowing me to set up these adjustments over and over again. (All chiropractic students worldwide feel the pain and commiserate with you). [Don't worry, no patients were harmed during the photography for this book and they were all subluxation-free afterwards!]

PREFACE

In order to be an effective and successful chiropractor, males and females alike must develop both a foundation of technical adjusting skills and also a deep understanding of key elements critical to achieving chiropractic technique success. I wrote this book to provide the petite practitioner a framework for additional manual manipulative skills, paying special attention to the differences in biomechanics. Being a petite female myself (63 inches, 115 pounds), I have a unique perspective on how to successfully treat patients of all shapes and sizes without sacrificing quality care, and to remain injury-free and enjoy a long career. In the following pages I will provide both new adjustment techniques as well as adaptive modifications to existing techniques that better fit the petite frame.

This text outlines specific step-by-step instructions and photographic depictions of how to provide the most biomechanically effective manual manipulations while staying injury-free as a chiropractic provider. Short video demonstrations of each adjustment are also provided online at www.HowToAdjust.com for concept clarification and technique execution. This manual also includes adaptive adjustment procedures for special population groups including: overweight patients, very muscular patients, and very tall patients.

This text is to be used only by trained and qualified professionals in the chiropractic and other professional manual manipulation fields or students of those trades. This book is not intended to replace careful instruction by qualified chiropractic physicians, but rather to serve as an adjunct to the foundational principles in chiropractic technique supplied by licensed instructors.

Chapter 1

Cervical & Cervicothoracic Junction

While the cervical region of the spine may not be notorious for posing particular challenges when employing manual manipulation, this chapter identifies one additional technique that employs less cervical rotation and limits extension, thereby increasing patient comfort and decreasing potential for adverse side effects of cervical manual manipulation.[1] There are many patients who may be treated using an inordinate amount of rotational torque accompanied by extension to their cervical spines due to ligamentous hyperflexibility, where slight modifications in technique eliminate the need for this, as demonstrated in the techniques within this chapter.

The cervicothoracic junction can be difficult to adjust due to the transitioning spinal curve from cervical lordosis to thoracic kyphosis. Most techniques involve powering through the surrounding soft tissues and applying a fair amount of torque and tension on the patient's head. This manner of adjustment technique can cause strain on the soft tissues and discomfort for the patient. In this section, I address three different techniques that help to avoid this while using both the patient and practitioner's biomechanics to your advantage.

The cervicothoracic junction should always be properly assessed when there is subjective complaint in either the cervical, thoracic, or upper extremity regions, and with special attention when encountering acute torticollis, as many incidences of such stem from spasmodic musculature and aberrant motion in this region of the spine.

Addressing soft tissue adhesions prior to the adjustment promotes comfort for the patient both during the adjustment and in the recovery period. This aids in restoring range of motion and decreasing nerve irritation.

Adjustment Techniques

"Ah, Flex It – Now Push It Real Good"

The cervical spine is well covered in other texts and is not uniquely challenging for the petite practitioner. However, the petite patient, as well as the elderly or arthritic patient, may need some slight modifications to the most commonly applied techniques. I use the following method which limits the amount of rotation and eliminates extension to the cervical spine and uses a gentle nudge rather than a high velocity thrust. Even patients who are apprehensive to manual manipulation of their neck are often open to this particular method because it is gentle, less dynamic, and limits rotation.

I seem to attract many patients to my practice who initially refuse cervical manipulation after having negative experiences in the past with other chiropractors, but after gaining trust with the patient through thorough examination, report of findings, and soft tissue work, almost all of them are willing to try manual manipulation. In performing soft tissue work with the patient in the supine position, you can get the adjustment set up and then ask them if they are okay with a little pulse of pressure from this position and voilà, they have already been adjusted without apprehension. [You're now on your way to becoming a chironinja!]. When you have been in practice for any length of time, you inevitably will encounter the patient who inquires about what they've seen in the action movies–a cervical adjustment looks a lot like a neck breaking Hollywood martial arts move. I always assure them that although I am freakishly strong for my size, I probably couldn't break their neck even if I tried, and I promise I'm not trying to.

By laterally flexing the patient's neck over your contact hand first, you can limit rotation and the need for a high velocity thrust. Let the patient's head remain resting on the headrest in the neutral position. Use a proximal interphalangeal (PIP) contact on your index finger, and use your non-contact hand to cradle the opposite side of the patient's head with your fingers straddling their ear, laterally flex the patient's neck over your contact hand until you feel the beginning of your end-feel, then add the least amount of rotation needed in order to lock the segment into end-feel and pulse lightly following the line of the patient's chin.

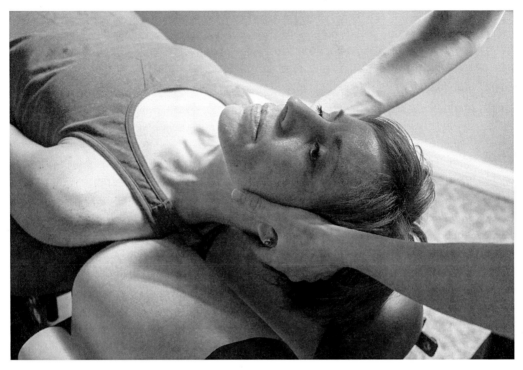

Image 1

Doctor Position:	Seated or standing in squatting athletic stance
Patient Position:	Supine
Contact Hand:	PIP on articular pillar of involved segment or an alternative thumb-pad contact
Non-Contact Hand:	First and second fingers straddling patient's ear, thumb on their face (avoid poking them in the eye)
Line of Drive:	Through the trajectory that follows the patient's chin
Thrust:	Minimal amount of force applied, just enough to gap the joint, a pulse about ¼ inch deep

☙

"Take A Seat"

I developed this adjustment technique while in school as a student. After struggling with adjustments in the cervicothoracic junction from day one with no success, even after receiving extra instruction from fabulous teachers, I realized that what I lacked was the speed, coordination, and upper body strength to successfully perform any of the techniques that were being taught to me. What I was good at however, after enduring endless hours of lectures, was sitting. As a sort of last-ditch effort and joke with one of my instructors, I thought, "What if I just sit on my patient since I clearly lack the biomechanical advantage here?" Amazingly, it worked! I thought it was a lucky fluke, but when many of my fellow classmates were struggling with the same thing, I offered my help and found this technique to be very reproducible and effective. This is my go-to technique for addressing joint restrictions in the cervicothoracic junction because it is so easy on my body.

> **Clinical Pearl**
> *When encountering patients experiencing episodes of acute acquired torticollis, this adjustment technique is favorable over others because it eliminates rotational torque and lateral flexion, which increases comfort for the patient who has significant range of motion restriction.*
> ☙

In clinical practice, when there is a family member observing in the room, I find this to be a perfect opportunity to make a silly joke or, at the very least, to comment that it looks more aggressive than it feels. This adjustment is best utilized for upper thoracic rotational and lateral flexion malpositions and doesn't require any torque on the patient's head. It uses the doctor's body weight with a fully extended contact arm to minimize stress on the shoulder for both the patient and the doctor.

It is especially helpful to have the patient drop their arm to the floor on the affected side with palm facing up, so that the doctor can then place their foot on the arm-rest for added leverage during the thrust in which you feign sitting on your contact hand.

With the patient prone, place a pisiform contact on the transverse process of the rotated upper thoracic segment. Keeping the contact arm locked in extension, step forward so that your contact hand is just behind you. The thrust occurs as your load is transferred through your locked elbow as you bend your knees in a sitting motion. This technique does require some practice and coordination.

This is the technique that I utilize most often for this region of the spine because it requires relatively little effort or strength from me and is also completely passive for the patient. My goals in practice are to be effective and excellent at my job and to still have enough energy after a long busy day at the office to go home and play with my young son and exercise as desired, remaining injury-free. This adjustment allows me to protect my shoulders and conserve some energy and is generally much more comfortable for the patient than the customary techniques involving lateral flexion of the head. Everyone wins!

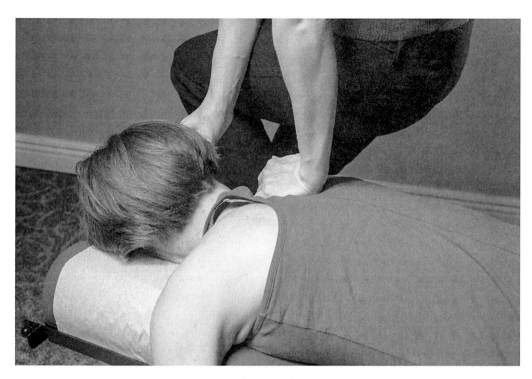

Image 2

Doctor Position:	Standing on the ipsilateral side as the listing, facing towards the patient's head, place your foot that is nearest the patient on the armrest and step forward so that with your arm fully extended, your contact hand is just behind your ipsilateral ischium
Patient Position:	Prone with ipsilateral arm extended towards the floor and palm facing up
Contact Hand:	Pisiform on the transverse process of the affected segment
Non-Contact Hand:	On the patient's head for stabilizing, with little to no pressure. (The patient's head is not laterally flexed during this adjustment and no pressure or thrust is applied with the non-contact hand).
Line of Drive:	Posterior to anterior
Thrust:	Keeping the arm of your contact hand extended, quickly bend your knees as if to sit on your contact hand as the patient achieves full exhalation

☙

"Double Fist Pump"

This is an awesome variation for the awkward areas of the CT junction encompassing the upper thoracic segments. Due to the minimal amount of force required during the thrust, this technique works great on older individuals and on patients with a hyperkyphotic thoracic curve or those with a Dowager's hump. In fact, the segments often move on pre-stress when employing this technique. This positioning allows you to keep your wrists in a neutral position, and when effective tissue pull is employed, minimal force is needed to make the adjustment happen successfully.

This technique utilizes your body weight (no matter how slight your build) to gently nudge the segments back home and doesn't require much physical effort, saving that for the next patient of the day who may require more effort and/or physical exertion. (We will address that later). Hesitant patients seem to like this variation as well because it doesn't require any lateral flexion of the head or torque.

Stand at the head of the table and make a fist with each hand. Place your fists on each side of the spinous process so that the metacarpal phalangeal joint (MCP) of the index fingers is in contact with the transverse processes (TPs) of the desired segment. Draw tissue slack in the I-S direction and, with a microbend in the elbows and neutral wrists lean into the patient as they breathe out, applying an impulse in the P-A direction as the patient achieves full exhalation.

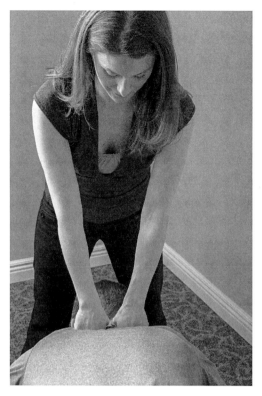
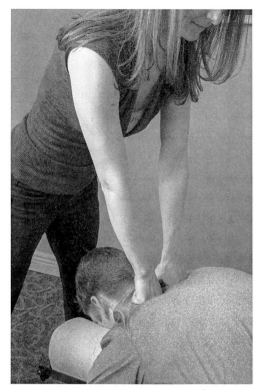

Image 3   *Image 4*

Doctor Position:	Standing at the head of the table facing towards the patient's feet (caudad)
Patient Position:	Prone
Contact Hands:	A fist is made with each hand and placed on each side of the spinous process over the TP of desired segment
Line of Drive:	P to A and I to S
Thrust:	Through the line of your first and second knuckles, as the patient breathes out, apply an impulse about ½ - 1 inch deep by leaning your body weight over your contacts (more depth for the larger or more muscular patient, less for the petite or arthritic patient)

"Iron Cross"

This adjustment is laid out nicely in some other texts, but this puts a different flare on it to make it easier on the practitioner's body while using biomechanics to your advantage. In other texts, the doctor stands beside the patient facing cephalically and uses the force of crossed arms through the pectoral region, causing strain on the shoulders and leaving the door open to injury.

In this variation, the doctor stands at the patient's head, facing caudally, and is able to keep their arms straight, leaning their body weight into the patient rather than applying a thrust using their shoulders and pecs.

Stand at the head of the table facing the patient's feet. With a hypothenar contact, place your contact hand on the TP of the desired segment. The noncontact hand will support and distract the patient's head, giving your hands a criss-crossed appearance. The thrust is employed as the patient exhales by leaning your body weight into your contact hand while applying distraction with slight lateral flexion away from the contact hand via the non-contact hand.

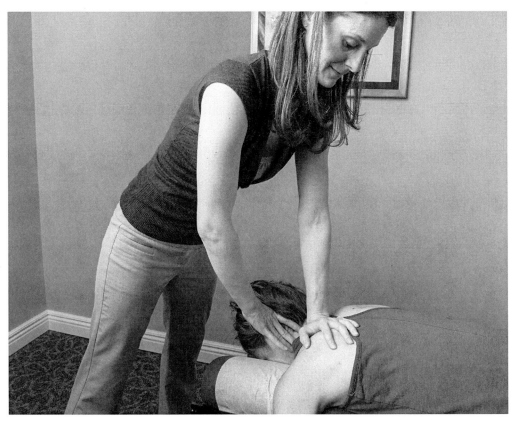

Image 5

Doctor Position:	Standing at the head of the table facing towards the patient's feet (caudad)
Patient Position:	Prone Contact
Hand:	Hypothenar contact using the opposite hand of the patient's involved side
Non-Contact Hand:	Web contact on side of patient's head, causing distraction in lateral flexion
Line of Drive:	P to A with slight distraction and lateral flexion of the patient's head.
Thrust:	Into the table as if to go through the patient's body as the patient exhales

Chapter 2

Thoracic

his region of the spine is typically the easiest to address because the plane of the facet joints allows for straight posterior to anterior pressure being used for most of the segments, which doesn't require a great deal of specialized technique regardless of the practitioner's body size. However, care must still be taken to avoid injury of the wrist, especially when adjusting very muscular or overweight patients, as it is commonplace to exert more force in these situations. Remember that brute force is not the only means to a successful adjustment, by adding finesse through ideal patient positioning and increased speed, the desired result can be achieved with less mass involved.

Some of the challenges facing petite chiropractors affect this region of the spine because there isn't always the weight behind the thrust to achieve a cavitation, nor the height to tower over the patient in order to drop your body weight during the employment of the thrust.

In this chapter, I introduce techniques that address these issues and employ careful body positioning and speed rather than brute force.

Adjustment Techniques

"Everyone Needs a Hug"

This is a variation of a popular thoracic adjustment with special attention to female anatomy and biomechanics both from the perspective of the practitioner and the patient. While this adjustment was taught to me in chiropractic school, I always had a difficult time working around the fact that I was essentially placing my breasts near my patient's face and laying on top of them, which, let's be honest, is just plain awkward. And from the patient perspective I always felt as though the doctor was smashing my breasts and arms and using a lot of weight and force where it wasn't crucial in order to achieve the desired result.

By placing a rolled towel between the patient's body and their crossed arms, this gives a little extra cushioning and an additional barrier between the doctor and patient. While the patient takes a deep inhale, I lower my body including my face below the level of their arms toward their feet to avoid that intimate feeling of laying on top of the patient with my breasts smashed up against them. Then as they exhale slowly and completely, I can use my shoulder on the same side as my contact hand to move their elbows apart to better position the patient and avoid getting myself jabbed in the sternum or neck by a pointy elbow *[Image 8]*.

This adjustment is especially helpful for muscular or overweight patients because it uses the patient's weight in addition to the doctor's weight on pre-stress. In these specific patient groups, additional leverage can be gained by floating your leg above the patient's body *[Image 9]*.

I have also found it to be especially useful when a misplaced rib head is complicating the aberrant motion of a thoracic spinal segment.

The patient begins in a seated position, and a thoracic board is placed on the table while you locate the aberrant segment. Using a twisting motion of your fist to place a thenar contact directly over the transverse process *[Image 6]*, the patient lies supine with arms crossed, their involved arm reaches for the contralateral shoulder, and the opposite arm reaches underneath the first for the opposite shoulder. Stand on the same side as the listing, rather than on the opposite side, as is the traditional method for this adjustment.

From this position, you eliminate the need to reach completely around the patient, which was challenging in itself for me, never mind if the patient was a large male, I simply couldn't provide any thrust from the traditional position of standing on the opposite side of the listing and then reaching over and around them. Standing on the same side as the listing also helps you avoid leaning your entire body across the chest of the patient, again limiting the intimacy of the traditional method.

Using this modification, you also have control over trunk motion by using the patient's elbows so that you can gain optimum biomechanical advantage with your contact hand directly under the greatest amount of weight and your non-contact hand approximating as if to squish the affected segment between your hands.

> **Clinical Pearl**
> *It may be helpful in difficult cases to also suspend your leg over the patient's body without making contact for extra dynamic movement.*
> ∞

Begin in a lunged position below (caudad to) the crossed elbows and as the patient inhales and then exhales, rise up over the patient's crossed elbows to approximate your hands on either side of the patient A to P, using your shoulder of the non-contact hand as necessary to separate the patient's elbows in order to avoid the patient's elbows hitting your sternum or throat *[Image 8]*. As the patient reaches near full exhalation, bend your knees and provide a thrust A to P while using your body weight to lean into the patient.

For lower thoracic segments that you attempt to adjust using this technique, it can also be helpful to ask the patient to tuck their chin as if to do a small sit-up, which helps to drive more of the patient's body weight caudally. In using this modification, your thrust also needs to be adjusted from straight A to P pressure to include I to S pressure simultaneously.

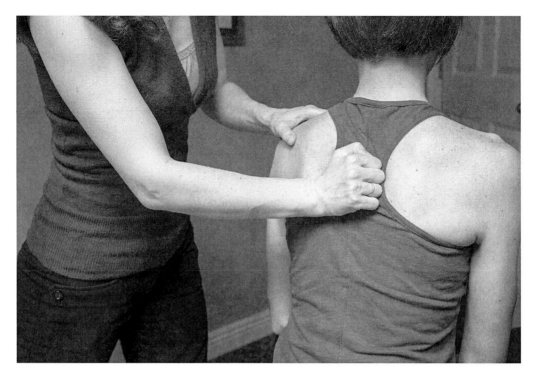

Image 6

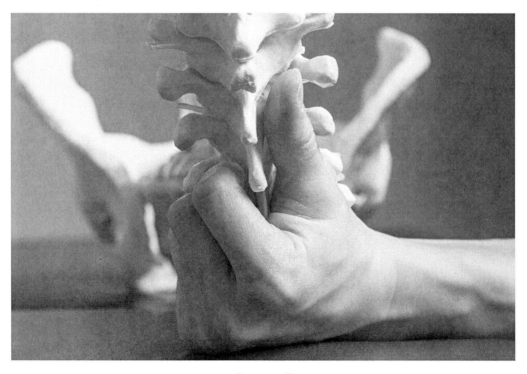

Image 7

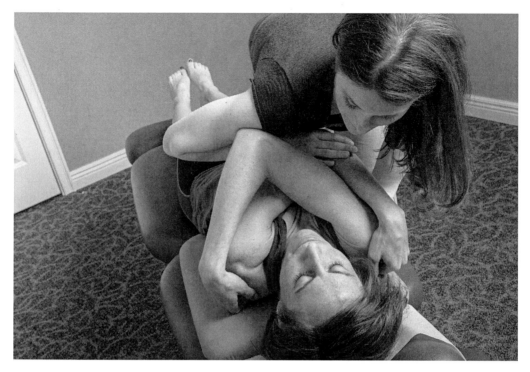

Image 8

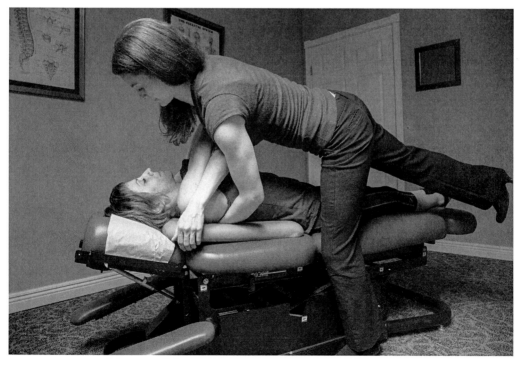

Image 9

Doctor Position:	Standing on the affected side, beginning below (caudad to) the patient's crossed elbows in a lunged position
Patient Position:	Supine with hand of affected side reaching for the opposite shoulder and other arm reaching underneath the first for the opposite shoulder with elbows approximated
Contact Hand:	Loose fist with thenar contact on the transverse process and spinous process falls in the depression where your fingertips meet your palm *[Image 7]*
Non-Contact Hand:	On patient's most anterior elbow, approximating your contact hand during the thrust
Line of Drive:	A to P with slight I to S
Thrust:	Using your inertia, as the patient exhales, bend your knees and lean your body weight over your contact

☙

"Tuck & Tumble"

I usually reserve this technique for when all my other usual techniques are inadequate to achieve the desired restoration of intersegmental joint motion, though it is gentle enough to use routinely and some practitioners even use it exclusively for adjusting the thoracic region. This technique seems to be a foolproof method to open up the thoracic cage and easily restore any lost motion into the thoracic spine by rotating the scapulas out of the way and spreading the rib cage apart.

By having the patient tuck their arms underneath them in the prone position, the practitioner maintains optimum biomechanics while the patient remains relaxed and comfortable. Patients find this particular technique to be gentle enough that they sometimes prefer it over the anterior method used in "Everyone Needs a Hug."

With the arms tucked underneath the patient, you achieve the same type of posture in opening up the thoracic cage as in the anterior method with arms reaching for opposing shoulders, but here you do so without adding their body weight into the equation, thus generating less passive pressure, which allows for added patient comfort.

With the patient prone, ask them to tuck their arms under their chest with flat hands and help them to tuck their elbows in. Apply your thrust with preferred contact(s) P to A and I to S. I use double knife-edge contacts for this adjustment to get a more specific contact on the transverse processes, but it works just as well with other hand contacts. Use the patient's exhalation of breath to ride down the spongy thoracic region, applying consistent pressure as the patient breathes out, then deliver a thrust as the patient achieves full exhalation.

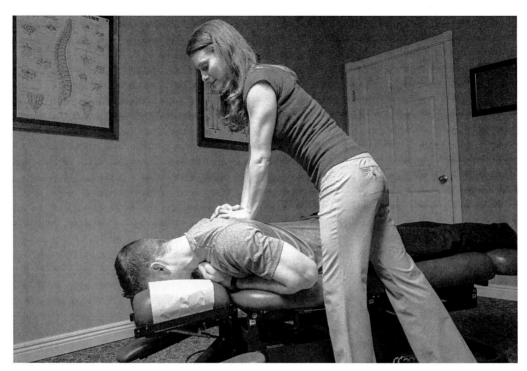

Image 10

Patient Position:	Prone with arms bent and tucked under them, elbows tucked in
Doctor Position:	Standing beside the patient with athletic stance
Contact Hands:	Double knife-edge (or other preferred contact)
Line of Drive:	P to A and I to S
Thrust:	Quick and shallow, about ½ inch of depth as the patient achieves full exhalation

❧

"Knife Thrower"

This adjustment is clearly laid out in other texts, but it is used as a non-specific, general mobilization, whereas I use a slight variation on the contact points to keep it segment specific. As a chiropractic patient myself, I sometimes find that prone, broad-contact thoracic adjustments feel heavy handed, as if the practitioner is on the verge of either breaking my ribs or grabbing my breasts from the side. Using the double knife-edge contact eliminates the latter issue and also helps the practitioner gain more advantageous biomechanics for themselves in keeping the wrists neutral without excessive, repeated hyperextension. Shifting your weight to the patient's midline and getting your body below your point of contact allows for a more advantageous position to deliver a good thrust. Rather than standing directly above your contact, as in other texts, which opens the door to pectoral strain, shoulder injury, and compromises the neutral alignment of the wrists.

I know many chiropractors with chronic wrist issues who benefit from changing their thoracic adjusting to using solely this method because it emphasizes proper biomechanics of the wrist. Having your body position slightly more caudal also enables the practitioner to deliver a dynamic thrust with arms straight to transfer the load of the force applied through your entire upper extremity and into the upper body without causing strain on the wrist or other joints in the chain.

With double knife-edge contacts and fingers interlaced, place the pisiforms on the desired TPs and drag tissue slack I to S. Center your chest to hover over the midline of the patient directly over your contacts. As the patient takes a deep inhale and then full exhale, apply light consistent pressure as you ride down towards the table to avoid recoil from the rib cage. Once full exhalation is reached and before the patient feels the impulse to inhale again, apply a thrust P to A with a rocking or scooping motion I to S.

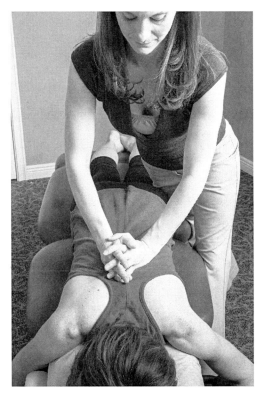 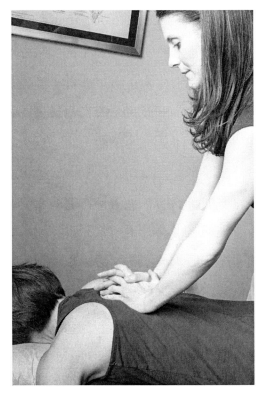

Image 11   *Image 12*

Doctor Position:	Standing on either side of the patient and slightly caudal, with weight shifted over the patient's midline to the best you are able
Patient Position:	Prone
Contact Hands:	Double knife-edge contacts, fingers interlaced, with pisiform located over TP of desired segment
Line of Drive:	P to A and slightly I to S
Thrust:	Deep and fast upon the patient's full exhalation. Sometimes in stubborn cases, it may even be helpful to actually let your feet leave the ground, putting all of your dynamic weight into the adjustment

"Don't Pop the Collar"

This slight variation of the previous technique addresses the upper thoracic segments where interlaced fingers may get in the way of the cervical spine, exerting unwelcome extension force on the neck of the patient. In this technique, the practitioner utilizes the same double knife-edge contact, but keeps the fingers in the laminar line on either sides of the spinous processes, which allows for the spinous process of C7 to duck underneath the spinous process of T1, alleviating some of the extension stress on the patient's neck.

With the patient prone and their arms extended toward the ground, stand on either side of the patient with weight shifted over their midline as much as possible. Contact the TPs of the desired segment using double knife-edge contacts and rest your fingers in the laminar line along the sides of the spinous processes and allowing fingers to flare out a bit near the cervical spine if needed in order to avoid contact with the patient's neck and to decrease cervical extension. The thrust is employed as the patient breathes out, P to A and slightly I to S with a quick, shallow movement.

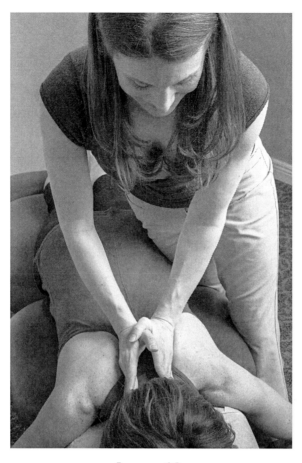

Image 13

Doctor Position:	Standing on either side of the patient and slightly caudal, with weight shifted over the patient's midline to the best you are able
Patient Position:	Prone, arms extended towards the floor
Contact Hands:	Double knife-edge contacts, with pisiform located over TP of desired segment and fingers resting on either side of the spinous process, thumbs crossed for added control
Line of Drive:	P to A and slightly I to S while the patient exhales
Thrust:	Quick and shallow

Chapter 3

Thoracolumbar Junction

This region of the spine gets a bad reputation for being a difficult area to adjust due to the transitioning curvature from thoracic kyphosis to lumbar lordosis. As the plane of the facet joints changes, proper positioning is elemental in achieving success with gapping the joint(s) while keeping the adjustment relatively comfortable for the patient. I have found that the upper segments of this region are best addressed in the prone position, while the lower segments are usually best addressed in the side-lying position. There was a definite gap in region specific instruction in this area for me during my time in chiropractic school, but this region demands its own techniques rather than lumping either the thoracic or lumbar techniques with the thoracolumbar region. This area is commonly overlooked during assessment, perhaps because is it difficult to adjust. Addressing issues in this region of the spine can relieve not only region specific pain, but also referred pain from the autonomic nervous system, specifically the digestive system and sexual organs.[2]

In this section, I cover techniques that make adjusting this region more accessible to the doctor and also more comfortable for the patient through variations of patient positioning and detailed descriptions of biomechanics to help achieve the optimal conditions for success in adjusting the thoracolumbar junction.

Adjustment Techniques
"Shoot for the Moon"

The typical suggestion and method of adjusting the thoracolumbar junction on a prone patient is with suspended inspiration. I don't know about you, but I always felt like someone was trying to knock the wind out of me when they tried that method, and the adjustment was rarely successful anyway. This technique outlines a much more comfortable way of adjusting the thoracolumbar junction, and I have found it to be more effective too!

There is nothing so mystical about this region of the spine that calls for such drastic change in customary methods of adjusting that we couldn't just use the typical "take a deep breath, breathe all the way out" preparation for the patient's body. The orientation of the laminar line and the joint plane do not necessarily dictate that suspended inspiration is better or even warranted. However, the typical P to A vector of force does not achieve the proper biomechanics to gap the joint(s), therefore, by adding a significant amount of I to S pre-stress and thrust, we can achieve an adjustment that is both comfortable for our patients and greatly effective.

This adjustment technique for the thoracolumbar junction employs a lot of I to S pressure, but with full exhalation rather than suspended inspiration, which keeps it more comfortable for the patient. When assessing the thoracolumbar junction, segments between T9 and T11 with flexion malposition, rotational restriction, or lateral flexion malposition are best treated using this technique.*

Standing in a lunge position with as much of your body directly over the patient as possible, using a double knife-edge contact, as the patient reaches full exhale, thrust P to A employing a lot of I to S directional force. After the first attempt, if you don't achieve the desired result, try again with more speed and pressure and make sure to engage your abdominal muscles, tightening your belly to concentrate your strength and force through your core.

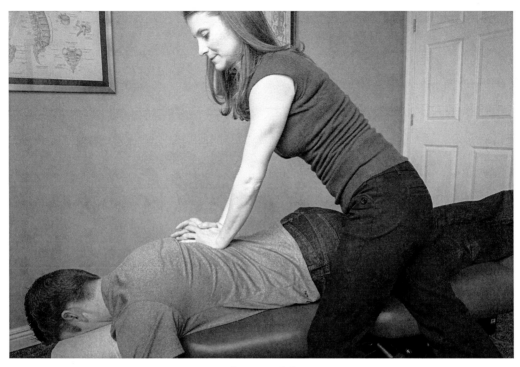

Image 14

Doctor Position:	Standing more caudad than for a typical thoracic adjustment with center of gravity shifted low
Patient Position:	Prone
Contact Hands:	Double knife-edge contacts
Line of Drive:	P to A and significant I to S
Thrust:	Towards the patients head, fast, and almost as if scooping upwards when the patient fully exhales

଼ଷ

*The lower segments from T12-L1 are best addressed with the next technique.

"Ring 'em Out"

The lower thoracic and upper lumbar segments can also pose technical challenges in adjusting and are often overlooked. Again, this region should be properly assessed when there are autonomic correlations to musculoskeletal symptoms, especially involving the reproductive and digestive systems. The segments from T12-L1 can be uncomfortable when adjusted P to A, even when using the previous technique, so placing the patient in side posture and isolating the segment(s) with additional flexion of the patient's hip alleviates most discomfort otherwise encountered in other techniques.

The other secret to effective and comfortable manual adjustment techniques in this area is to bring your contact hands close together with the aberrant segment in between them. This is achieved by placing your non-contact hand on the patient's arm and the patient arm resting low on their abdomen, as if to squish the involved segment between your hands. Employing the kick-start method of thrust is usually the most effective in this region because it allows for fast speed and contributes to rotational force, which both attribute to success when adjusting the lower thoracic and upper lumbar segments.

With the patient laying on their side, grab the wrist of the arm that is down against the table and pull their upper body towards you so that they are laying on their scapula *[Image 15]*. Then with your cephalad leg against the table for stability, bend the patient's top leg so that their knee is bent enough to tuck their toes behind the knee of the bottom leg.

Next, change your body position to face the patient's head with your hip against the table for stability. Reach your contact hand around the patient's pelvis, hooking underneath the iliac crest, with your non-contact hand grab under their top knee, lifting and pulling the patient's body toward the edge of the table and down toward their feet at the same time *[Image 16]*.

This enables you to properly position them so that their shoulder isn't jammed into the headrest, they are close enough to the edge of the table not to obstruct your thrust by their leg hitting the table, and puts your body close to theirs for better leverage and patient security

Flex the patient's knee toward their chin as much as needed until you are able to feel the motioning of the desired segment or, alternatively, until you achieve endfeel. Place your knee in the crease of their bent top knee *[Image 17]* and initiate a downward kick, while simultaneously pulling with your contact hand and applying sacral distraction with your elbow.

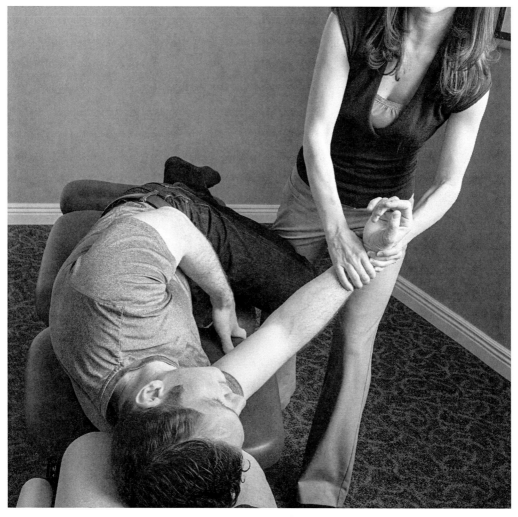

Image 15

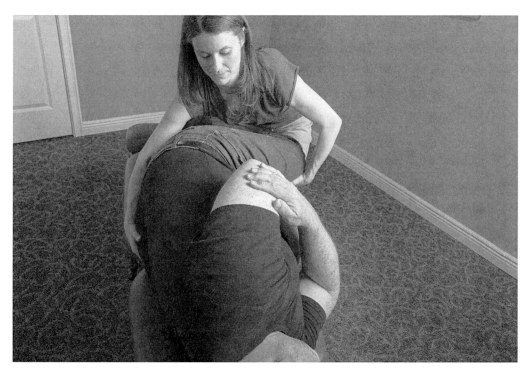
Image 16

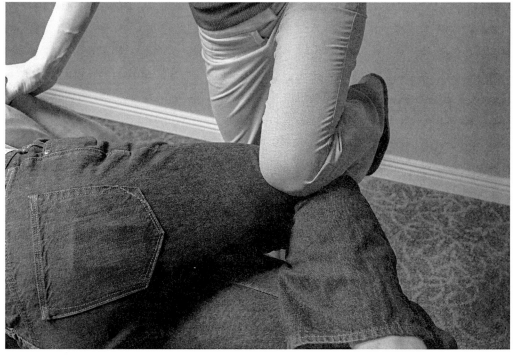
Image 17

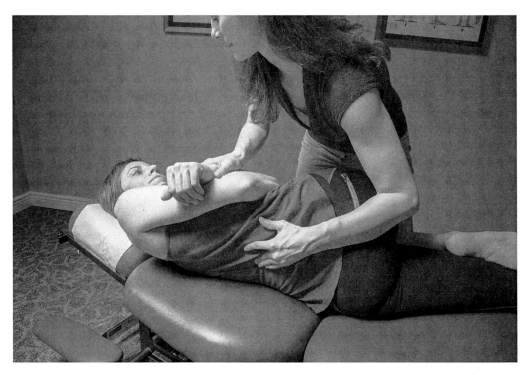

Image 18

Doctor Position:	Standing with your body anchored against the table, using the kickstart method with your knee placed on the patient's bent knee
Patient Position:	Side-lying with top leg bent to 90 degrees and toes of top leg tucked behind the knee of the other leg
Contact Hand:	Digit contact on involved spinous process with forearm applying sacral distraction
Non-Contact Hand:	Placed on patient's crossed arms, with counter pressure applied from A to P towards the involved segment as if to squish the segment between your hands
Line of Drive:	Through the patient's abdomen, towards your body and a downward kick of the leg
Thrust:	Quick combination of downward pressure on the leg, rotational pull on the desired segment, and distraction using the forearm

Chapter 4

Lumbar & Pelvis

Before beginning chiropractic school I wondered about my physical ability to effectively perform lumbar side posture adjustments, mostly due to my petite size. Having small hands, being height challenged, and/or having a petite frame does not inherently inhibit you from attaining the ability to effectively achieve lumbar side posture adjustments, even on overweight or especially muscular patients.

The trick is speed, finesse, and maintaining optimal biomechanics to avoid injuring your shoulder, wrist, or lower back. This region is notorious for causing injury amongst chiropractors[3] for compromising the practitioner's body mechanics while these injuries may be prevented by changing a few key aspects of body positioning for both the patient and the practitioner.

> **Clinical Pearl**
> *When there is a marked amount of soft tissue spasm, tenderness, or otherwise increased tissue turgor at or around the level of L3, the psoas muscle should also be assessed and appropriate therapeutic techniques applied.*
> ଓ

One of my favorite clinical scenerios is when a patient looks at my petite size and wonders if I am physically capable of alleviating their lower back pain, and then after the adjustment says with surprise and disbelief in thier voice "Wow, you're a beast, I feel better already!" I've been told over and over again that even linebacker sized men weren't able to deliver effective adjustments to their lower back, but I seem to do it with ease.

Most petite practitioners struggle with adjusting this region because we are taught to "drop weight," "climb up," or "lean over" our patients. All of these actions can pose anatomic challenges and compromise our biomechanics. In this chapter, I describe how to overcome these anatomic challenges while using your biomechanics to your advantage.

In this area, like most others, it is advantageous to first address soft tissue adhesions, which will make achieving intersegmental motion easier. Careful patient positioning is key to achieving both patient comfort and optimal biomechanics. Especially for the acute patient where it can be more difficult to achieve optimal patient positioning, it is imperative that the doctor use every aspect of their biomechanics to their advantage.

In traditional methods of adjusting the lumbar region in side posture, the noncontact hand is placed on the patient's shoulder which automatically moves your energy out away from the point of the adjustment, causing a biomechanical disadvantage [Image 19].

By placing the patient's arms lower on the torso and being careful not to place any extra pressure on the non-contact hand, squishing the involved segment between your contact points avoids the doctor getting too stretched out themselves and limits trunk rotation to achieve a more precise adjustment at the desired segment.

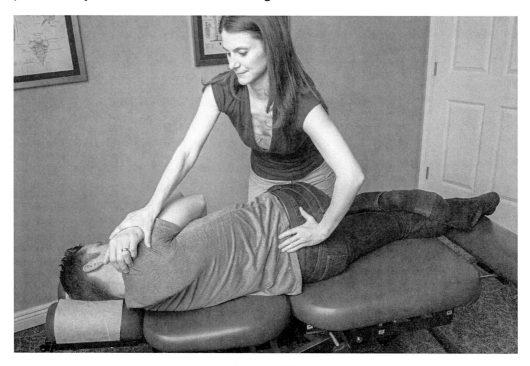

Image 19

Adjustment Techniques

"The Lumbar Lambada"

It seems like everyone struggles with manual adjustment techniques for the lumbar spine, regardless of gender, height, weight, etc. First of all, there is a lot of tissue to feel through in order to find the joint restrictions, and then having to work through all of that tissue, (which often is hypertonic), poses significant barriers. Addressing the soft tissue is a key element, not to be overlooked, but this text is about the actual adjustment, not instruction on physiological therapeutics, therefore, address this as you see fit as the practitioner.

Moving on, I was significantly challenged here by my short stature, and I don't have body mass to throw around either. I also can't reach over and around my patients' bodies like someone with longer arms can. However, I was able to find a way to achieve my desired results consistently by properly positioning the patient and by using my own biomechanics to the best of my ability. Basic elements that are commonly overlooked include rolling the patient toward you, lifting your leg up to meet the patient's body when necessary, and leaning your body against the table to stabilize your balance and prevent the patient from rolling too far. Lean in close to the patient to use physics to your advantage so as not to create a long lever with your arm extended around the patient's body. This also helps aid in relaxation for the patient and helps them trust that you won't let them roll or drop them off of the table.

Encourage your patient to let their belly relax, which is traditionally achieved by having the patient take a deep breath in and exhaling; however, I have found that telling the patient to "let your belly relax" or "let your belly go" is much more effective in attaining a more relaxed demeanor from the patient. Wait to deliver your thrust until the moment you feel the patient relax their belly and they are no longer holding increased abdominal pressure, which is usually felt at the exact moment that there is additional rotation in the patient's trunk when you have them in a locked out position. Apply your thrust at this precise moment and you will be successful in your attempt to gain intersegmental motion.

Using a digit contact on the lamina of the affected segment while using your forearm for pelvic/sacral distraction, maintain neutral wrist alignment and keep your elbow close to your side *[Image 20]*. This hand placement can be used with either a kick-start *[Image 21]* or traditional side posture adjustment style *[Image 22]*. The distraction that your forearm provides, allows the segments to gap much more easily, thus making intersegmental motion easier to achieve. Approximate your hands, virtually squishing the desired segment to limit upper trunk rotation and to isolate the specific desired segment. When utilizing the kickstart method, make sure to kick down, not back, in order to further initiate specific segmental rotation.

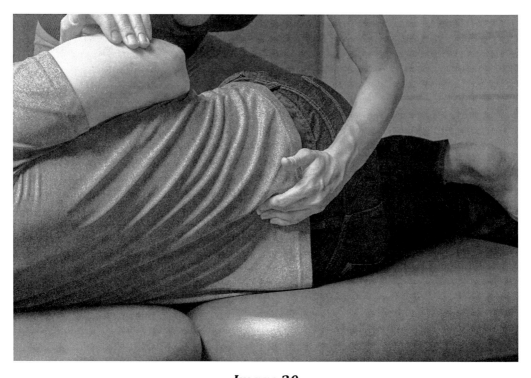

Image 20

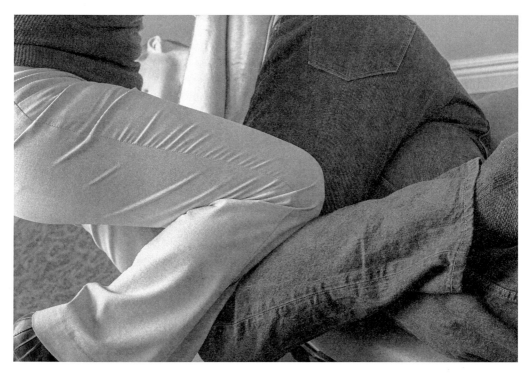

Image 21

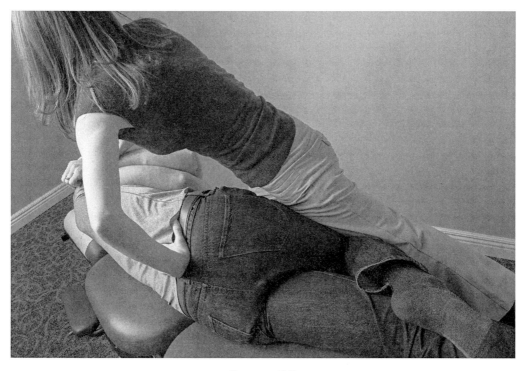

Image 22

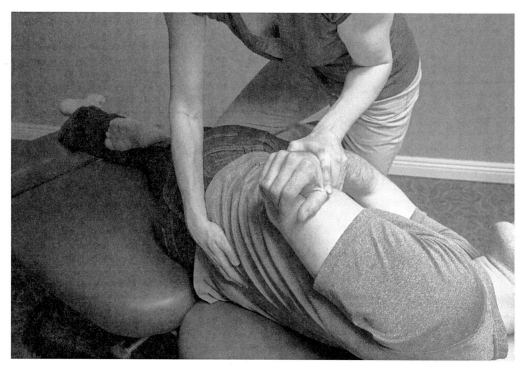

Image 23

Doctor Position:	Standing with your cephalad thigh against the table and your caudad knee contacting the patient's bent top knee
Patient Position:	Side-lying Contact Hand: Digit contact on the desired segment with forearm distracting the sacrum
Non-Contact Hand:	On the patient's wrist over their abdomen, approximating your contact hand
Line of Drive:	Squish your hands together to squeeze the desired segment between your hands
Thrust:	Kick your leg down towards the ground as if to start a motorcycle

"The Elvis"

This adjustment isn't as fool-proof as the "Lumbar Lambada", but it works nicely on smaller patients or more flexible patients and allows less strain on your body. This technique allows the practitioner to keep their body more upright rather than leaning over the patient, which is especially useful for practitioners who are prone to or are recovering from injuries to the lower back and shoulder.

Throughout chiropractic school, I was always told to lean over the patient and drop my body weight to achieve the desired thrusting force, which my short height and small stature don't allow for and the force required from that body position put a lot of strain on my shoulder. It is no secret that a lot of chiropractic students and DCs early in their careers end up with disabling injuries within the first five years of practice.[4] Using this technique, you limit the amount of strain on your shoulder and lower back because your body position remains erect and lateral to the patient, and most of the thrusting force comes from the action of your leg rather than your shoulder.

To apply this technique, keep your elbow in close to your body and don't lean over the patient too far staying low and vertical instead. The thrusting motion is similar to the trademark dance moves of Elvis, hence the name, with one foot staying planted while the other leg does all the action (referred to as the action leg).

Using a thenar contact on the lamina of the affected segment, position the patient in side posture. The tibial tuberosity of the patient's bent knee is your contact point for your action leg. Position your caudad leg's inner thigh just distal to the knee on the patient's tibial tuberosity. Your non-contact hand is on the patient's forearm, same as for the "Lumbar Lambada". The thrust occurs as simultaneous movements: a push using your contact hand to initiate lumbar rotation and a swift lateral to medial push with your knee of the action leg to facilitate distraction and lumbar flexion. Speed is especially important using this maneuver, and your feet stay planted eliciting a pivot movement with the foot of the action leg.

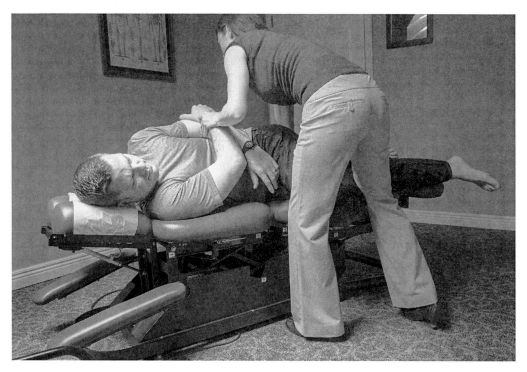

Image 24

Doctor Position:	Standing with your cephalad leg against the table, your caudad leg contacts the tibial tuberosity of the patient's bent knee with either the medial side of your knee or lower inner thigh
Patient Position:	Side-lying Contact Hand: Thenar contact on the lamina of the desired segment with straight and neutral wrist, may apply sacral distraction with forearm
Non-Contact Hand:	On patient's wrist over their abdomen
Line of Drive:	Pivot your caudad foot to swiftly move your knee medially while pulling your contact hand anteriorly
Thrust:	Shallow and quick with coordinated movement

☙

Chapter 5

Extraspinal

This section is not meant to be an exhaustive list of extremity adjustments, but rather an adjunct to your knowledge base on the subject just as the rest of this text is intended to be.

In this section I provide some new modifications of adjustments that add comfort for the patient and are more favorable to the biomechanics of the petite practitioner. Some of these techniques can be self-applied and are useful in relieving any physical issues that the practitioner may experience after long, busy days/weeks of practicing manual manipulation.

Adjustment Techniques

"Hitchhiking Together"

I have found that restrictions of the proximal joint of the thumb commonly cause impingement syndromes where patients present with localized pain and/or referred pain to the wrist or distally into the thumb. The typical recommendation for adjusting this joint is to apply long axis distraction with a downward force on the thumb, which is not always effective at gapping the joint and can cause discomfort for the patient, especially if there is inflammation and/or arthritis in the joint. Instead, I apply a squeezing pressure, rather than a common forceful thrust, which gaps the joint gently, allowing the thumb to move freely once again.

Clinical Pearl
You can even perform this adjustment on yourself!
ଓ

Seated beside the patient on their involved side, reach your adjacent arm over the patient's arm and interlace your fingers with theirs, keeping your thumb on the outside of theirs. With a web contact at the anatomical snuffbox, squeeze your thumb and index finger together as if to scoop the patient's thumb away from their wrist.

The true clinical pearl with this adjustment technique is that you can perform this adjustment on yourself, which is especially helpful to the practitioner who utilizes manual soft tissue methods in their practice. When this joint becomes jammed, we can lose grip strength, have thumb and/or wrist pain, and sometimes paresthesias. Taking good care of your hands is vital to having a long career in the chiropractic profession, as our hands are our most important tools.

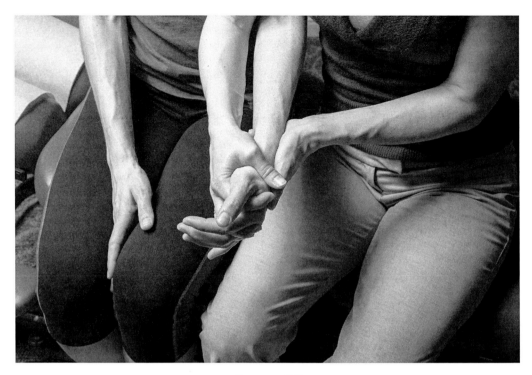

Image 25

Doctor Position:	Seated beside the patient on their involved side
Patient Position:	Seated with arm relaxed
Contact Hand:	Interlace fingers with the patient using their involved side and your hand opposite theirs (ie patient right hand, doctor left hand); web contact where the patient's thumb meets their wrist in the anatomical snuffbox
Non-Contact Hand:	None needed, but you may support the patient's wrist from beneath as shown in the above image
Line of Drive:	Proximal to distal, lifting the thumb away from the wrist
Thrust:	Squeeze

"Thumb Wrestling"

This joint often gets jammed in people who work with their hands and the customary rotational adjustment for the distal interphalangeal joint doesn't work very well here. I started using this adjustment because I utilize a lot of soft tissue work in my practice using my hands, and I naturally wanted to do the opposite action to undo the jamming of the joint when my body was feeling it after a long, busy day.

Grasp the distal end of the patient's thumb with your index DIP under the pad of the thumb and your thumb pad covering the patient's entire distal thumb joint. Flex to almost 90 degrees, firmly pinching while distracting the joint. The thrust is a gentle lift of the patient's distal thumb away from the rest of their hand.

This adjustment is also useful for practitioners to use on themselves, especially after employing a great deal of manual soft tissue techniques in practice, which is jamming to the distal thumb joint.

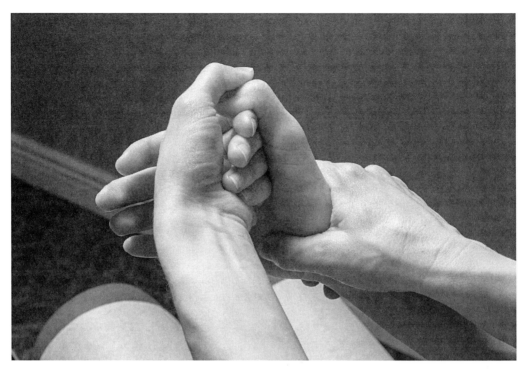

Image 26

Doctor Position:	Seated or standing so that you can attain the proper angle to grasp the thumb of the patient
Patient Position:	Arm of involved hand relaxed and arm outstretched either seated, standing, or laying supine
Contact Hand:	First middle phalynx butted up against the patient's distal interphalangeal joint line and thumb covering the nail and whole distal phalynx flexing it to 90 degrees
Non-Contact Hand:	Grasping the patient's wrist or none
Line of Drive:	Distract the joint pulling the distal phalynx away from the patient's hand
Thrust:	Slow and steady distraction, increasing until the joint gaps

"Bunny Hop"

This adjustment is great for generalized and non-descript knee pain, especially when all orthopedic tests are negative and even when advanced imaging fails to identify anything abnormal. I treat a lot of athletes in my practice and encounter a lot of cases of such knee pain. In some cases it is point specific, other times it is generalized knee pain, and sometimes the pain moves from one point to another. In nearly all cases, this adjustment is helpful, essentially providing general distraction of the tibial-femoral joint with the knee in a slightly flexed position and initiating glide of the tibia anteriorly. Obviously, thorough examination needs to be performed prior to manual manipulation, especially to rule out ACL or patellar tendon tear or rupture, in which case this technique would be contraindicated.

With the patient supine, have the patient drape their affected leg off the side of the table. Bend the patient's knee to about a 90 degree angle and grasp all fingers of both hands behind the patient's calf in the depression between the two heads of the gastrocnemius muscle with bilateral thumbs on either side of the tibial tuberosity. Position your legs on either side of the patient's knee contacting the patient's mid-calf on both sides with the medial distal thigh at the attachment of the vastus medialis muscle.

The doctor checks the joint play and initiates any slight internal or external rotation of the tibia as indicated. The practitioner then bends their knees and as you pull the tibia anteriorly, hop backwards as you straighten your knees while the patient's knee remains bent in slight flexion.

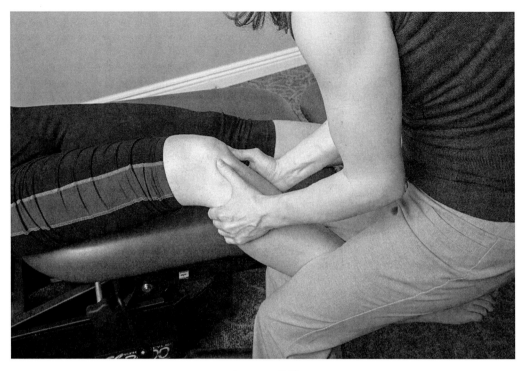

Image 27

Doctor Position: Standing beside the table on the patient's affected side with knees bent and distal medial thighs contacting either side of the patient's mid-calf

Patient Position: Supine with affected leg draped off the side of the table and foot dangled so that it is not contacting the floor

Contact Hands: Wrapping around the patient's proximal calf with fingers meeting in the midline where the two heads of the gastrocnemius separate and thumbs on either side of the tibial tuberosity

Line of Drive: P to A

Thrust: Initiated from a small hop backwards as you straighten your knees and pull anteriorly with your hands

"Mini Hop"

This adjustment for the cuboid is both gentle and effective, isolating the desired joint and maintaining firm contact on the ankle while feeling very comfortable for the patient. It is especially helpful when treating acute and chronic lateral ankle sprains. This adjustment, in combination with long axis distraction of the talus, will address most general ankle complaints.

Traditional methods of adjusting this area of the ankle can be non-specific and require brute force from the upper body for the thrust, but this method utilizes straight arms and the addition of a mini hop with the patient's ankle grasped between the knees of the practitioner, which greatly diminishes any strain on the practitioner's body.

Standing at the foot of the table with the patient supine, grasp the involved ankle using a thenar contact on the dorsal cuboid and fingers wrapping around the ankle. Bring the patient's ankle between your knees and bend your knees a little. Extend the patient's leg while straightening your knees and hopping backwards a little bit, pushing down with your contact hand.

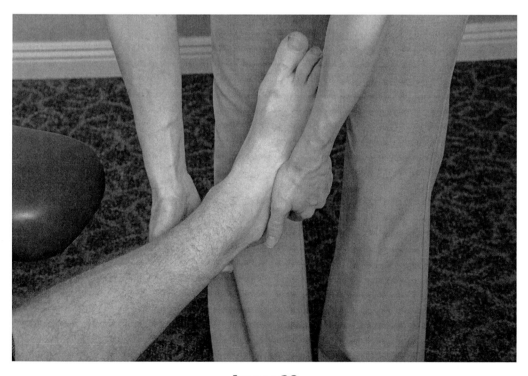

Image 28

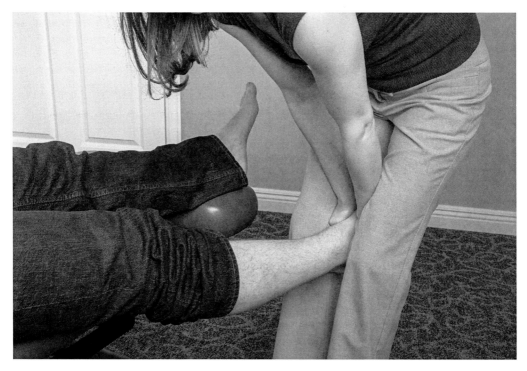

Image 29

Doctor Position:	Standing at the patient's feet with knees bent slightly
Patient Position:	Supine with affected ankle draped off the side of the table
Contact Hands:	Thenar (or alternative bilateral thumbs) on dorsal aspect of the cuboid, fingers wrapping firmly around the ankle
Line of Drive:	S to I
Thrust:	Distraction of the joint in a long axis with an impulse from the hands caudally

Chapter 6

Adjusting The Overweight Patient, The Very Tall Patient, & The Very Muscular Patient

Patients falling into these specific populations of body composition can be particularly challenging for the petite practitioner. By utilizing the techniques already laid out in this text, you will be successful with manual manipulative therapy in such patients most of the time. This section covers general considerations for biomechanics and positioning, both for the patient and for the practitioner.

One of the first questions I asked myself before starting chiropractic school was, "What if a 300-pound man walks into my office with low back pain? Am I physically capable of adjusting him?" The answer is, absolutely! You just have to use proper biomechanics and use physics to your advantage. Using some soft tissue work to prime the pump doesn't hurt either. When I first began in private practice, I often deferred to using a drop piece on overweight patients or large men, but as I developed these modifications in addition to using the other techniques laid out in this manual, I found that I was very seldom using my drop piece as I have complete confidence that even on a 300+-pound man, manual side posture adjustments are easily attainable and effective.

General considerations for the overweight population are that their bodies will take up more space; they are closer to the ceiling when laying prone, they are higher on the table when laying on their side, and trying to reach around their bodies for anterior thoracic or lumbar side posture adjustments becomes more challenging for a petite practitioner with smaller arm span. Don't be afraid to get your body into the most advantageous position for you to make the adjustment happen, even if that means kneeling on the table beside your patient during prone thoracic adjustments or hiking your leg up to be parallel with the ground for side posture adjustments.

When treating very tall patients, there are more of the patient's appendages in the way when the patient is side lying. In this instance, proper patient positioning is essential so that their leg doesn't contact the table, which stops your thrust, and also so that their knee or foot doesn't contact the floor. Their arms may be too long to use a rolled towel for an anterior thoracic adjustment as previously described for "Everyone Needs a Hug", and in this case I have them hug a bolster *[Image 30]*.

Arms may also get in the way during side posture adjustments, but don't be tempted to place your non-contact hand on their shoulder, as this will create too much displaced leverage for the your body mechanics and also encourages more generalized trunk rotation for the patient, which makes achieving specific intersegmental motion more difficult. You may have to stand somewhat further back from the table during side posture in order to use the patellar knee contact, as long as you are firm with your contact hand and contact knee, the patient will not over-rotate to fall on the floor.

In working with especially muscular patients such as body builders, there is a lot more hypertonic tissue to work through, both for proper assessment and during the adjustment. There is also more likely to be a rebound effect from the thrust where the practitioner feels as though the patient's body bounces them away without achieving the desired adjustment. These issues can be addressed by some pre-emptive soft tissue therapy, the practitioner tightening the abdominal muscles during thrusting, and proper patient positioning.

In this chapter, there are a few additional variations of techniques for typically challenging areas to adjust on these types of patients. Recall the previous techniques also and employ them as well for this subset of patients. Where additional challenges are faced, the following techniques are helpful.

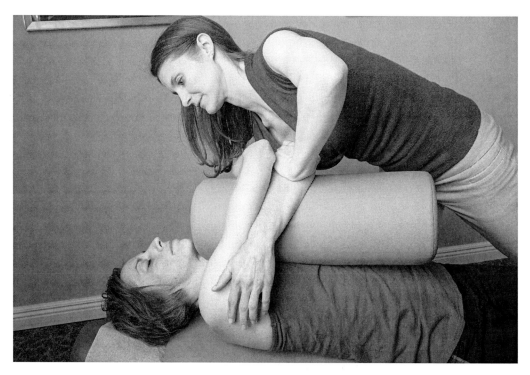

Image 30

Adjustment Techniques

"Fire Hydrant"

Working with the larger patient body type, often you will encounter decreased flexibility and increased tissue turgor. These factors can work to your advantage if you pay attention. Lumbar side posture is often challenging in this subset of patient body types, but it doesn't have to be. Patient positioning is critical to making your body's biomechanics work for you. Again, in many cases there will be decreased flexibility in general, which equates here to decreased lumbar rotation and the patient's limited ability to flex their hip with the knee bent in side posture.

This adjustment is also useful in the patient presenting with acute lower back pain with significantly decreased range of motion due to pain. In that case, allowing the patient to remain as comfortable as possible by eliminating too much pre-stress tension aids in their ability to relax enough to allow for a smooth and easy adjustment. As an extra clinical pearl, I always adjust the more painful side first in these cases so that the patient doesn't tense up in apprehension for what they know is coming next.

> **Clinical Pearl:**
> In the patient presenting with acute lower back pain, adjust the most painful side first. This way, the patient is less likely to tense up in apprehension.
> ☙

Place the patient in side posture with their arm that is down on the table drawn towards you so that the patient is laying on their scapula rather than their humerus. Because the patient's body will take up more space due to larger size, their bent knee will also be higher off the ground than it typically is, to combat this, press down on the patient's bent knee to bring it closer to the floor and hike up your leg to meet theirs, positioning your inferior patellar pole inside the crease of the patient's bent knee. Contact the lamina of the desired segment with the distal pad of the middle finger, keeping your elbow in close to your body to limit the chance of shoulder strain.

Then guide the patient's body through lumbar flexion as you move your knee with theirs to find the point of greatest intersegmental restriction. Rotate as much as necessary to achieve end-feel by applying increasing pressure with your contact knee and simultaneously pulling on the lamina of the desired segment toward you, which usually in this population doesn't require much rotation, employ the kick-start adjustment, kicking your contact knee down towards the ground. The thrust is quick and forceful, but typically doesn't have to be deep due to the patient's limited flexibility. When properly positioned and pre-stress tension is applied, the additional lumbar rotation achieved through the thrust is not necessary to be extremely dynamic.

It is also helpful for the practitioner to tighten their abdominal muscles during the thrust for further concentrated force and to avoid the chance for self-inflicted lower back stress.

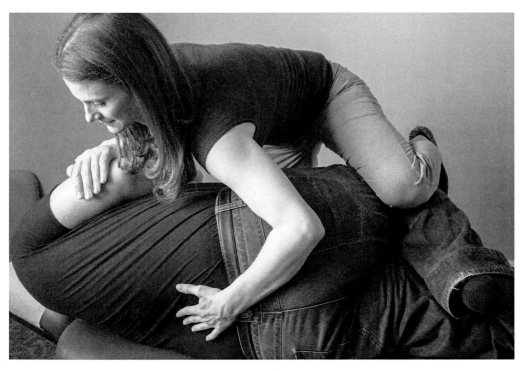

Image 31

Doctor Position:	Standing with your cephalad leg against the table for stability, your caudad leg becomes your contact knee by placing your tibial tuberosity in the crease of the patient's bent top leg
Patient Position:	Side-lying with top leg bent and foot hooked behind the opposite knee
Contact Hand:	Digit contact on the lamina of the affected segment
Non-Contact Hand:	Firmly applying counter-pressure on the patient's crossed forearms
Line of Drive:	P to A with rotation towards the doctor
Thrust:	Swift, hard kick down with a firm digit pull deep through the patient's torso

ଓ

"Wrestling Match"

I sometimes joke with patients that I am a chiropractor during the week and a professional wrestler on the weekends. And I have been known to joke about putting elastic rebound ropes around the perimeter of my treatment rooms as are present in a wrestling ring. But all jokes aside, that extreme isn't necessary to achieve effective manual manipulation on large or very muscular patients. I have had very satisfied patients call me all kinds of nicknames–"chiro-ninja," "beast," "warrior," "magician," and the list goes on. I don't take offense to these terms because I know that my patients are only stating their confidence in my ability to get the job done.

The thoracic region may traditionally be fairly easy to adjust, but in the overweight and very muscular patient, this area can be challenging. When adjusting a large or overweight patient, I often need to get up on my tip toes in order to compensate for the lost height above my contact points due to their body sitting higher off the table *[Image 32]*. Alternatively, don't be afraid to climb up on the table if you don't have a pneumatic elevation table or your table just doesn't get low enough.

Place the knee of your non-dominant side on the table next to the patient's torso and get your body positioned over the patient's midline as best you can *[Image 33]*. Lean your whole body into the thrust and get as dynamic as necessary.

I usually try to use the least amount of force necessary for every adjustment I do, often times thrusting twice in quick succession to achieve both responsive muscle twitch relaxation from the patient and utilizing a deeper, more forceful thrust on the second attempt. If the patient's body seems to bounce you right off of your contact, you aren't centered over them enough and are too low, so don't be afraid to get your knee up on the table next to the patient in order to get a little higher up and more centered.

Get up on your tip toes and lean your thigh into their body so that you are positioned directly over the patient and slightly more caudal than the involved segment. As you thrust with double knife-edge contacts, keep your arms straight with a microbend in the elbows. Bend your knees quickly to rock your torso down perpendicular to the prone patient while leaning your body weight into them. If you don't achieve your desired result on the first try, you can use a successive thrust, but you have to account for their body's inertia to rock back inferiorly before you can thrust I to S again.

If the patient is very high toward the ceiling or especially muscular, I will sometimes even jump a little, letting both feet leave the ground to drive my thrust into the patient *[Image 34]*. Just remember that in this case, it is important to keep your arms straight with a microbend in your elbows in order to avoid wrist and/or shoulder injury.

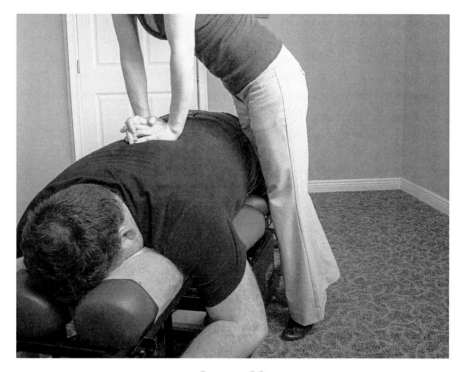

Image 32

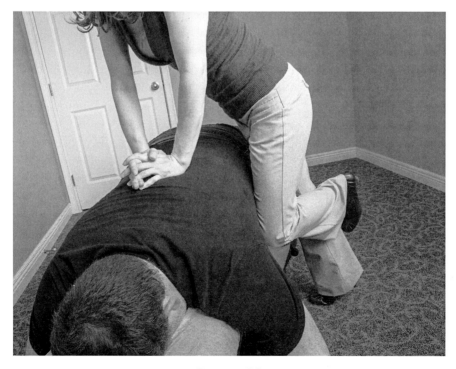

Image 33

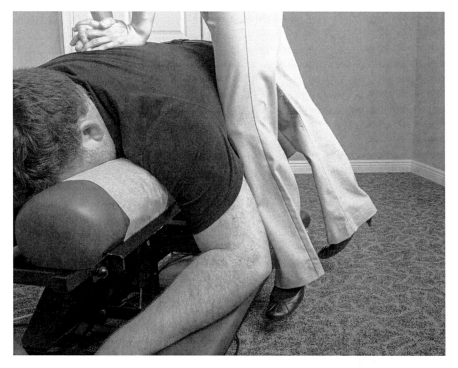

Image 34

Doctor Position:	Standing on tip toes with thigh leaning against the patient's side, or with knee of opposite leg on the table beside the patient as pictured in Image 2
Patient Position:	Prone with table as low to the ground as you can get it
Contact Hands:	Double knife-edge
Line of Drive:	P to A and I to S
Thrust:	Dynamic and forceful

☙

"No-Neck Nunchucks"

The larger the person, the more tissue, which in the cervical region often equates to difficulty in palpating all seven individual segments of the spine for joint play. Many practitioners resort to a generalized motioning of the cervical spine known commonly as the "cervical break". Achieving a specific adjustment is even more difficult, but using a thumb contact helps with precision and specificity. When there is increased tissue turgor and excessive amounts of tissue in the cervical region, it is imperative to properly assess the lost mechanics of motion at each segment in order to determine line of drive.

To do this, don't be afraid to move tissue out of the way as necessary, including reaching in between skin folds or rolls as needed. I recommend palpating using a thumb-pad contact in these circumstances, which then sets you up nicely for the adjustment as well so that you can just thrust on the segment as you find the restrictions. It is not as easy to just employ intersegmental rotation here for the thrust, because of the perceived decreased space between segments due to added tissue. The lower the cervical segment, the more the line of drive shifts to be toward the patient's contralateral shoulder, and the higher the listing, the more the line of drive shifts to be through the line of the patient's eyes.

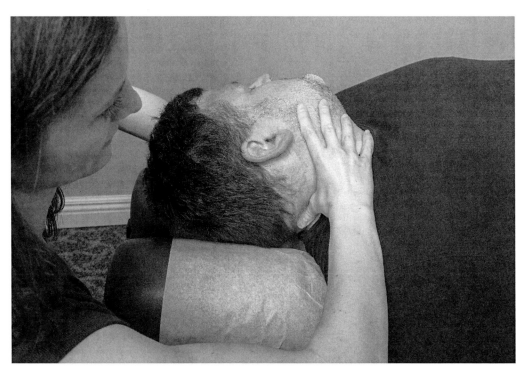

Image 35

Doctor Position:	Squatting in athletic stance with elbow of contact hand close to side and contralateral elbow raised in 90 degree bend (not limp)
Patient Position:	Supine
Contact Hand:	Thumb pad on the desired segment with fingers resting lightly on the patient's face, taking care not to poke them in the eye
Non-Contact Hand:	First and second fingers straddling the ear and the rest of the hand cradling the head
Line of Drive:	Through the line of the patient's shoulders for lower segments C5-7, through the line of the patient's chin for C3-4, and through the line of the patient's eyes for upper segments C1-2
Thrust:	Quick motion as if to move through the patient's neck and thrust out the other side

Appendix

Definitions and abbreviations

P   =   posterior

A   =   anterior

I   =   inferior

S   =   superior

TP   =   transverse process

PIP   =   proximal interphalangeal joint

DIP   =   distal interphalangeal joint

SP   =   spinous process

Knife-edge   =   outermost edge of the fifth metacarpal

Thenar   =   fat pad of the palm along the first metacarpal

Hypothenar   =   fat pad of the palm along the fifth metacarpal

CT   =   cervicothoracic

TL   =   thoracolumbar

References

1. Haneline M, Lewkovitch G. Chiropractic manipulation and cervical artery dissection. JACA. 2007 Jan/Feb;20-26.

2. Leboeuf-Yde C, Pedersen EN, Bryner P, et al. Self-reported nonmuskuloskeletal responses to chiropractic intervention:a multination survey. J Manipulative Physiol Ther. 2005 Jun;28(5):294-302.

3. Holm SM, Rose KA. Work-related injuries of doctors of chiropractic in the United States. J Manipulative Physiol Ther. 2006 Sep;29(7):518-23.

4. Kuehnel E, Beatty A, Gleberzon B. An intercollegiate comparison of prevalence of injuries among students during technique class from five chiropractic colleges throughout the world: a preliminary retrospective study. J Can Chiropr Assoc. 2008 Aug;52(3):169-174.